Gluten-Free Living

Healthy Gluten-Free Diet Slow Cooker Recipes

Janet Cook

DISCLAIMER

All rights reserved. No part of this publication or the information in it may be quoted from or reproduced in any form by means such as printing, scanning, photocopying, or otherwise without prior written permission of the copyright holder.

Disclaimer and Terms of Use: Effort has been made to ensure that the information in this book is accurate and complete. However, the author and the publisher do not warrant the accuracy of the information, text, and graphics contained within the book due to the rapidly changing nature of science, research, known and unknown facts and internet. The Author and the publisher do not hold any responsibility for errors, omissions or contrary interpretation of the subject matter herein. This book is presented solely for motivational and informational purposes only.

New to Gluten-Free Diet?

Check out my book Gluten-Free Diet for beginners. It has all the information you need to start your diet plus lots of delicious everyday quick and easy recipes the whole family will love.

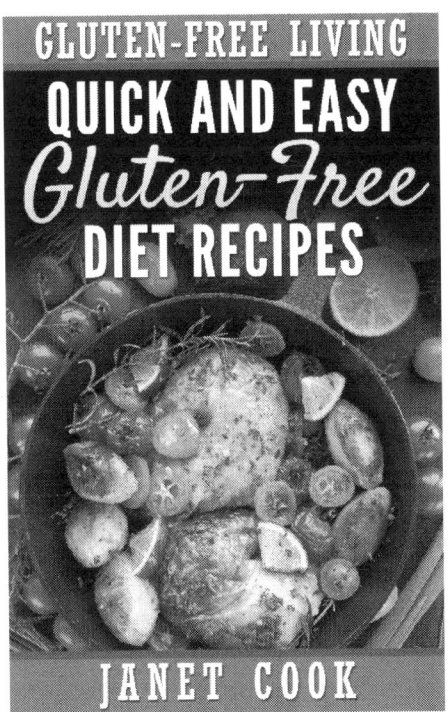

CONTENTS

DISCLAIMER 3
CONTENTS 7
INTRODUCTION 9
BREAKFAST RECIPES 11
   Nuts and Raisins Pudding 11
   Southern California Sausage, Beans, and Potatoes 13
   Cinnamon-Banana Oatmeal 15
   Ham with Green Peas 16
   Sunny Morning Omelet 17
   Pocket Bacon Breakfast 19
   Pineapple Gluten-Free Bread Pudding 21
LUNCH RECIPES 23
   Gluten-Free Chicken Tacos 23
   Crock Pot Gluten-Free Beefy Tomato Soup 25
   Crock Pot Chili Chicken 27
   Roasted Seasoned Quinoa 29
   Shredded Pork Tenderloin and Salad 31
   Tuna and Gluten-Free Tortilla Soup 33
   Spiced Balsamic Salad 35
   Meaty Gluten-Free Lasagna 37
   Gluten-Free Chicken Noodle Soup 39
DINNER RECIPES 41
   Rosemary Turkey Roast 41
   Sugar and Spice Chicken 43
   Corned Beef Tapa 45
   Barbecue Pork Roast with Green Beans 47

Creamy Cheesy Turkey Casserole 49

Cheese and Beef Meatballs 50

Juicy Lamb Chops 51

Korean-Style Honeyed Chicken 53

Turkey Soda Roast 55

Creamy Corn and Pork Bits 56

Peppery Creamy Chicken 57

Honey Mustard Pork Slices 58

Pork Chops and Buttered Vegetables 59

Vegetable and Legume Stew 61

Chili Salmon Fillets 63

Cheesy Beef Ravioli 65

DESSERT RECIPES 67

Vanilla and Honey Bananas 67

Cinnamon Pears 68

Spiced Up Veggies with Apples 69

Strawberry Fudge Slices 70

Caramel Apples 71

Almond Chocolate Drink 72

Pineapple Gluten-Free Bread Pudding 73

S'mores Squares 75

CONCLUSION 77

INTRODUCTION

In this day and age when everything has to be fast, efficient, and practical, food—one of the most important needs of life—is often overlooked. People tend to eat in a rush, favor premade foods over home-cooked meals, and sometimes can't even take the time to sit down for a meal. This may free up the time we need to meet the obligations of our career and interpersonal lives, but where has our health and wellness gone?

It doesn't have to be complicated to prepare quickly a meal that can be share with family or friends. All you need to do is place the ingredients in the slow cooker, start the cooking process and forget about it for a couple of hours. And voilà, you will have wonderful meal ready when you are and your home will smell so wonderful.

Cooking with a slow cooker is very convenient. It's makes amazing one pot meals that are healthy and delicious. These recipes are 100% gluten-free, made especially made, for people suffering from celiac disease, gluten intolerance, or for people who would like to start a gluten-free lifestyle and stay away from processed foods.

Sit back and enjoy. You are about to experience the best of Slow Cooker Gluten-Free Recipes.

BREAKFAST RECIPES

Nuts and Raisins Pudding

Servings: 6
Preparation time: 5 minutes
Cooking time: 3 hours

Ingredients:
¾ cup glutinous rice
¼ cup butter, melted
2 cups milk
½ cup chopped pecans
½ cup raisins
½ cup brown sugar
1 teaspoon cinnamon
½ teaspoon nutmeg

Directions:
- In the slow cooker, combine melted butter, then glutinous rice, then milk.
- Cook for 1 hour on high.
- Add nuts, raisins, brown sugar, cinnamon, and nutmeg. Continue cooking for another 2 hours.
- Slice into preferred sizes.

Nutrition facts per serving **(182 g)**
Calories: 352
Total fat: 14.9 g
Carbohydrates: 49.5 g
Dietary fiber: 0.5 g
Sugars: 24.8 g
Protein: 5.9 g

Southern California Sausage, Beans, and Potatoes

Servings: 6
Preparation time: 20 minutes
Cooking time: 5 hours

Ingredients:
1½ cups dried mung beans
1 pound pork sausage
5 cloves garlic, minced
1 medium yellow onion, diced
2 cups gluten-free chicken or vegetable stock
1 tablespoon turmeric
1 tablespoon chili powder
2 teaspoons dried rosemary
1 green bell pepper, chopped
1 red bell pepper, chopped
1 teaspoons cumin
1 pound potatoes, cubed
Salt and pepper to taste

Directions:
- Add 6 cups of water to a large saucepan. Add the beans and bring to a boil over high heat. Reduce heat to medium high, and let simmer for 15 minutes.
- Meanwhile, crumble the sausage in a frying pan and brown. Drain the fat. Add the garlic, and stir until fragrant.
- Chop the vegetables, and place in the slow cooker.

- Drain the beans and place in the slow cooker with the vegetables and the browned sausage mixture.
- Add the stock and all the remaining ingredients. Season with salt and pepper, and gently stir to combine. Cover and set the slow cooker on low heat. Cook for 7 hours on low. The beans should be fork tender.

***Nutrition facts per serving* (235 g)**
Calories: 371
Total fat: 33.5 g
Carbohydrates: 8.9 g
Dietary fiber: 1.8 g
Sugars: 1.3 g
Protein: 15.0 g

Cinnamon-Banana Oatmeal

Servings: 8
Preparation time: 5 minutes
Cooking time: 6 hours

Ingredients:
2 cups gluten-free oats
2 teaspoons cinnamon powder
4 medium-sized bananas, sliced
¼ cup brown sugar
¼ cup butter, melted
1 cup milk
½ teaspoon salt

Directions:
- Place butter, milk, and brown sugar in the slow cooker.
- Cook for 1 hour on low.
- Add in gluten-free oats, cinnamon powder, sliced bananas, and salt.
- Cook for another 5 hours.
- Sprinkle with more cinnamon before serving.

Nutrition facts per serving (224 g)
Calories: 168
Total fat: 2.8 g
Carbohydrates: 31.0 g
Dietary fiber: 4.4 g
Sugars: 3.4 g
Protein: 6.7 g

Ham with Green Peas

Servings: 6
Preparation time: 20 minutes
Cooking time: 8 hours

Ingredients:
3 cups cooked ham, diced
2 cup green peas, fresh or frozen
2 carrots, diced
3 red potatoes, diced
1 medium yellow onion, sliced
2 teaspoons gluten-free soy sauce
2 cups gluten-free chicken or vegetable broth
Salt and black pepper

Directions:
- Add all the ingredients to the slow cooker. Stir to mix well. Season with salt and pepper.
- Cook on low for 8 hours.

Nutrition facts per serving (325 g)
Calories: 301
Total fat: 3.0 g
Carbohydrates: 55.3 g
Dietary fiber: 8.5 g
Sugars: 4.6 g
Protein: 18.1 g

Sunny Morning Omelet

This is a great recipe to prepare before going to bed. It will be ready when you wake up!

Servings: 6-8
Preparation time: 15 minutes
Cooking time: 9 hours

Ingredients:
10 eggs
2 teaspoons dried basil
½ teaspoon garlic powder
8 slices precooked bacon, chopped
2 potatoes, diced
½ cup cheddar cheese, shredded
1 red bell pepper, diced
2 tomatoes, diced
1 medium-sized yellow onion, sliced
Salt and pepper

Directions:
- Add all the ingredients to the slow cooker, except the eggs. Stir to combine.
- Whisk the eggs, and pour over the prepared ingredients in the slow cooker.
- Cook on a low setting for 8-9 hours.
- Season with salt and pepper, and serve.

***Nutrition facts per serving* (280 g)**
Calories: 490
Total fat: 32.4 g
Carbohydrates: 21.5 g
Dietary fiber: 3.0 g
Sugars: 1.1 g
Protein: 25.9 g

Pocket Bacon Breakfast

Servings: 4-6
Preparation time: 15 minutes
Cooking time: 10 hours

Ingredients:

1 pound bacon, diced
¼ cup onion, diced
½ teaspoon fresh garlic, minced
2 tomatoes, diced
1 green or red bell pepper, diced
¼ cup cheddar cheese, grated
¼ cup parmesan cheese, grated
6 eggs
Salt and pepper

Directions:

- Layer the bacon, onion, garlic, tomatoes, and bell pepper at the bottom of the slow cooker.
- Cook on low for 5 hours.
- In a mixing bowl, whisk the eggs with cheddar and parmesan cheese. Place this mixture over the prepared ingredients in the slow cooker.
- Cook on low for another 5 hours.
- Season with salt and pepper to taste.

Nutrition facts per serving (175 g)
Calories: 492
Total fat: 28.6 g
Carbohydrates: 31.4 g
Dietary fiber: 2.7 g
Sugars: 2.7 g
Protein: 25.0 g

Pineapple Gluten-Free Bread Pudding

Servings: 6
Preparation time: 15 minutes
Cooking time: 6 hours

Ingredients:
1 cup pineapple, chopped into bite-sized chunks
3 tablespoons butter, melted
1 cup milk
¼ cup condensed milk
¼ cup brown sugar
1 tablespoon lemon juice
8 gluten-free bread slices, cut into cubes
3 eggs
1 teaspoon cinnamon

Directions:
- In the slow cooker, place butter, milk, condensed milk and brown sugar. Whip the eggs and place in the bottom layer too.
- Layer in the gluten-free bread slices then cook for 2 hours.
- Add the pineapples, lemon juice, and cinnamon.
- Cook for 4 hours on low.
- Slice into desired sizes.

***Nutrition facts per serving* (225 g)**
Calories: 547
Total fat: 17.2 g
Carbohydrates: 86.5 g
Dietary fiber: 2.5 g
Sugars: 49.2 g
Protein: 13.3 g

LUNCH RECIPES

Gluten-Free Chicken Tacos

Servings: 8
Preparation time: 5 minutes
Cooking time: 6 hours

Ingredients:
4 boneless chicken breasts, about 6 oz. each
2 tablespoons gluten-free taco seasoning
2 teaspoons dried oregano
1 teaspoon black pepper
2 cups chicken broth
1 medium onions, sliced
16-24 Gluten-free taco shells, soft or hard or a mix of both

Garnish
Shredded Tex Mex cheese mix
Red bell pepper, diced
Shredded iceberg lettuce
Guacamole
Fresh chopped cilantro

Directions:
- Place the chicken breasts in the slow cooker, and season with black pepper, taco seasoning, and oregano. Carefully add the chicken broth, and layer the onions on top.
- Set the slow cooker to high and cook for 6 hours.

- Remove the chicken breasts to a cutting board, and shred with two forks. Put the meat back into the broth to keep warm.
- Prepare the garnishes and place in serving bowls. Arrange the hard taco shells on a baking sheet and bake in the oven for 6-10 minutes at 350°F, until warm. If using soft taco shells, wrap them in aluminium foil before placing on the baking sheet.
- Place the warmed taco shells on a serving plate. Drain the chicken and serve with all the garnish ingredients. Let everyone create their own tacos.

Nutrition facts per serving (90 g)*
Calories: 74
Total fat: 1.8 g
Carbohydrates: 1.3 g
Dietary fiber: 2.1 g
Sugars: 0.5 g
Protein: 14.6 g

without garnish

Crock Pot Gluten-Free Beefy Tomato Soup

Servings: 6-8
Preparation time: 15 minutes
Cooking time: 3 hours

Ingredients:
2 pounds ground beef
2 cups beef stock
1 cup green lentils
1 cup black beans
½ cup GF creamed corn
1 can diced tomatoes, 28 oz
½ cup green bell pepper, diced
½ cup red bell pepper, diced
¼ cup prepared yellow mustard
¼ cup sour cream, to garnish
10 cherry tomatoes, to garnish
Salt and pepper to taste

Directions:
- In a frying pan, brown the ground beef and drain the fat. Add to the slow cooker, together with the stock, lentils, black beans, corn, canned tomatoes, mustard, green bell pepper, and red bell pepper.
- Cook on high for 1½ hours or low for 3½ hours. Garnish with sour cream and cherry tomatoes.

Nutrition facts per serving *
Calories: 489
Total fat: 26.9 g
Carbohydrates: 19.6 g
Dietary fiber: 14.1 g
Sugars: 12.5 g
Protein: 24.8 g

Crock Pot Chili Chicken

Servings: 4-5
Preparation time: 25 minutes
Cooking time: 7 hours

Ingredients:
4 teaspoons chili powder
½ cup red bell pepper
3 teaspoons oregano, ground
2 teaspoons turmeric, ground
1 cup tomato paste
½ cup tomato sauce
¼ cup minced garlic
¼ cup onion, diced
1 pound boneless chicken breast, diced
1 cup dried pinto beans, rinsed
Olive oil

Directions:
- Boil pinto beans for 8-10 minutes.
- In a large skillet, heat 2 tablespoons of olive oil on medium-high oil. Fry chicken on all sides for 2-3 minutes or until, golden brown.
- Drain, then put in the slow cooker together with chili powder, red bell pepper, ground oregano, ground turmeric, tomato paste, tomato sauce, mashed garlic, and diced onion.
- Cook for 7 to 9 hours on low.

***Nutrition facts per serving* (470 g)**
Calories: 645
Total fat: 32.0 g
Carbohydrates: 55.7 g
Dietary fiber: 20.9 g
Sugars: 13.4 g
Protein: 50.5 g

Roasted Seasoned Quinoa

Servings: 4-6
Preparation time: 30 minutes
Cooking time: 5 hours

Ingredients:
2 cups quinoa, rinsed
4 cups vegetable or chicken broth
2 tablespoons olive oil
1 tablespoon dried basil
½ tablespoon dried oregano
4 cloves garlic, minced
2 teaspoons grainy Dijon mustard
2 teaspoons honey
1 medium yellow onion, diced
Salt and freshly ground black pepper
Parsley, chopped, for serving

Directions:
- In the slow cooker, mix together quinoa, olive oil, broth, basil, oregano, garlic, onions.
- Season with salt and black pepper to taste.
- Cook for 5 hours on low.
- Serve garnished with chopped parsley.

Nutrition facts per serving (85 g)
Calories: 165
Total fat: 3.6 g
Carbohydrates: 8.3 g
Dietary fiber: 1.7 g
Sugars: 5.6 g
Protein: 1.4 g

Shredded Pork Tenderloin and Salad

Servings: 6-8
Preparation time: 30 minutes
Cooking time: 4 hours

Ingredients:
1 pound pork tenderloin
6 tablespoons olive oil, divided
¼ cup minced garlic
1 small onion, diced
2 teaspoons oregano, ground
½ cup red bell pepper, diced
½ cup green bell pepper, diced
¼ cup parmesan cheese, grated
1 small avocado, diced
6 cups mixed baby greens salad
1 tablespoon fresh parsley, chopped
½ cup tomatoes, diced
1 cucumber, chopped
3 teaspoons lemon juice
2 teaspoons honey
Salt and pepper

Directions:
- Place the pork, 3 tablespoons of olive oil, garlic, onion, oregano, red bell pepper, and green bell pepper in the slow cooker.
- Cook for 4 hours on low.
- To prepare the salad, mix together avocado, baby greens, parsley, tomatoes, and cucumber.

- To prepare the dressing, in a small mixing bowl whisk together 3 tablespoons of olive oil, parmesan cheese, lemon juice, and honey. Stir in the vegetables from the slow cooker, and season with salt and pepper. Pour over the salad, and mix to coat.
- Remove the pork to a cutting board, and shred with two forks.
- Divide the salad equally between plates. Top with the still-warm shredded pork.

***Nutrition facts per serving* (142 g)**
Calories: 299
Total fat: 12.8 g
Carbohydrates: 19.9 g
Dietary fiber: 2.7 g
Sugars: 1.7 g
Protein: 29.9 g

Tuna and Gluten-Free Tortilla Soup

Servings: 6
Preparation time: 15 minutes
Cooking time: 5 hours

Ingredients:

2 cups canned tuna, packed in oil, about 4 4 oz. can, drained
4 cups vegetable broth
1 cup tomato sauce
2 tomatoes, diced
1 small yellow onions, diced
3 cloves garlic, minced
1 bunch of parsley, chopped
2 teaspoons paprika
2 teaspoons ground cumin
2 teaspoons chili powder
1 ½ cup gluten-free tortillas chips, crushed
Salt and pepper

Directions:

- Add tuna, broth, tomato sauce, tomatoes, onions, garlic, parsley, paprika powder, cumin, chili powder to the slow cooker.
- Cook for 5 hours on low.
- Add crushed tortilla chips.
- Season with salt and pepper before serving.

***Nutrition facts per serving* (645 g)**

Calories: 390
Total fat: 21.0 g
Carbohydrates: 24.6 g
Dietary fiber: 7.4 g
Sugars: 11.1 g
Protein: 32.6 g

Spiced Balsamic Salad

Servings: 10
Preparation time: 10 minutes
Cooking time: 3 hours

Ingredients:
6 cups of balsamic vinegar
¼ cup brown sugar
½ cup lemon juice
2 teaspoons dried oregano
1 teaspoon ginger, grated
½ teaspoon black pepper
3 cups iceberg lettuce
3 cups romaine lettuce
2 carrots, shredded
Salt and freshly ground pepper

Directions:
- Place balsamic vinegar, brown sugar, lemon, oregano, ginger, and black pepper in the slow cooker.
- Cook on low for 3 hours.
- Place over iceberg lettuce, romaine lettuce and carrots.
- Top with dashes of salt and pepper before serving.

***Nutrition facts per serving* (215 g)**

Calories: 81
Total fat: 0.0 g
Carbohydrates: 17.1 g
Dietary fiber: 2.5 g
Sugars: 6.2 g
Protein: 0.3 g

Meaty Gluten-Free Lasagna

Servings: 4-6

Preparation time: 10 minutes
Cooking time: 6 hours

Ingredients:
1 pound ground beef
½ pound ground pork
1 small yellow onion, chopped
2 cloves garlic, minced
1 6 oz. can tomato paste
24 oz. tomato sauce (3 cups)
2 teaspoons Italian seasoning
Gluten-free lasagne noodles, cooked
1 cup mozzarella cheese, shredded

Directions:
- In a large skillet over medium-high heat, brown the ground beef and pork. Drain the fat. Add the onions and garlic and stir until fragrant, about 2 minutes. Remove from heat and stir in the tomato paste.
- In a measuring cup or bowl, mix the tomato sauce with the Italian seasoning.
- Layer in the slow cooker, ¾ cup of tomato sauce and 1/3 of the meat mixture. Cover with gluten-free lasagne, and repeat the same layers 2 times. Spoon the remaining tomato sauce on the top.
- Set the slow cooker on low heat and cook for 5 hours.

- Add the shredded mozzarella cheese, and cook for 1 more hour until the cheese is melted and the lasagne noodles are cooked.

***Nutrition facts per serving* (464 g)**

Calories: 1097
Total fat: 46.2 g
Carbohydrates: 93.0 g
Dietary fiber: 8.3 g
Sugars: 20.7 g
Protein: 78.7 g

Gluten-Free Chicken Noodle Soup

Servings: 6
Preparation time: 20 minutes
Cooking time: 8 hours

Ingredients:
1 pound rotisserie chicken, shredded
1 teaspoon salt
1 teaspoon black pepper, ground
7 cups chicken broth
1 cup potatoes, diced
1 stalks of celery, diced
1 carrot, diced
3 bay leaves
1 small onion, diced
2 teaspoons minced garlic
1 package of small shaped gluten-free noodles
4 eggs
Parsley, chopped for garnish

Directions:
- Season the chicken with salt and pepper.
- Arrange the chicken in the slow cooker and add the broth, potatoes, radishes, bay leaves, onion, and garlic.
- Cook on low for 5 hours.
- Whisk the eggs and add to the slow cooker, together with the gluten-free noodles.
- Cook for 3 more hours.
- Garnish with chopped parsley.

Nutrition facts per serving **(574 g)**

Calories: 465
Total fat: 27.0 g
Carbohydrates: 19.9 g
Dietary fiber: 2.5 g
Sugars: 2.6 g
Protein: 33.6 g

DINNER RECIPES

Rosemary Turkey Roast

Servings: 8
Preparation time: 10 minutes
Cooking time: 9 hours

Ingredients:
1 turkey, about 10 pounds
5 tablespoons butter, melted
5 tablespoons rosemary, ground
3 tablespoons oregano, ground
2 teaspoons black pepper, ground
1 cup chicken broth and more if required
1 bunch of parsley, chopped
½ teaspoon salt
2 teaspoons black pepper, whole

Directions:
- Rub turkey with rosemary, oregano, and ground black pepper.
- Place turkey in the slow cooker, and add butter, broth, salt, and whole black pepper.
- Cook for 9 hours on high.
- Check every hours, add chicken broth as needed
- Serve with boiled or baked potatoes, and salad.

Nutrition facts per serving **(246 g)**
Calories: 293
Total fat: 9.5 g
Carbohydrates: 2.8 g
Dietary fiber: 1.0 g
Sugars: 0.0 g
Protein: 49.6 g

Sugar and Spice Chicken

Servings: 6
Preparation time: 15 minutes
Cooking time: 8 hours

Ingredients:
1 large chicken, cut into serving pieces (or 6-8 pieces of chicken)
2 tablespoons honey
¼ cup brown sugar
5 teaspoons cinnamon
¼ cup butter, melted
2 tablespoons rosemary, ground
2 tablespoons oregano, ground
2 teaspoons chili powder
¼ cup garlic, minced
2 teaspoons black pepper, ground
1 cup chicken broth

Directions:
- In a small mixing bowl, combine sugar, cinnamon, rosemary, oregano, chili powder, and black pepper. Mix well, and rub on the chicken pieces. Place the pieces in the slow cooker.
- Stir together the honey, butter, garlic, and chicken broth, and carefully pour around the chicken pieces.
- Cook for 8 hours on low.

Nutrition facts per serving (235 g)

Calories: 485
Total fat: 22.1 g
Carbohydrates: 39.5 g
Dietary fiber: 0.3 g
Sugars: 38.7 g
Protein: 29.4 g

Corned Beef Tapa

Servings: 4-8
Preparation time: 10 minutes
Cooking time: 8 hours

Ingredients:
2 pounds cooked corned beef, shredded
3 tablespoons olive oil
1 cup Korean beef stew sauce
¼ cup onion, chopped
¼ cup garlic, minced
2 tablespoons oregano
1 tablespoon black pepper, whole
1 bunch parsley, chopped
¾ cup potatoes, diced
¾ cup carrots, diced
1 cup beef broth

Directions:
- In a large skillet, fry the shredded beef for 10-12 minutes, or until slightly crispy.
- In a slow cooker, combine the cooked beef, beef stew sauce, onion, garlic, oregano, black pepper, parsley, potatoes, carrots, and broth.
- Cook for 8 hours on low.
- Serve with steamed rice.

***Nutrition facts per serving* (1255 g)**

Calories: 955

Total fat: 43.3 g

Carbohydrates: 88.4 g

Dietary fiber: 24.1 g

Sugars: 28.0 g

Protein: 54.9 g

Barbecue Pork Roast with Green Beans

Servings: 4-6
Preparation time: 10 minutes
Cooking time: 7 hours

Ingredients:
2-3 pounds pound pork loin roast
2 teaspoons ground sage
4 teaspoons dried thyme
4 tablespoons olive oil
¾ cup barbecue sauce
½ cup chicken broth
2 pounds string green beans, trimmed and chopped in 1-inch pieces

Directions:
- Mix the olive oil with the sage and thyme.
- Pour the broth in the slow cooker, and add the pork.
- Brush the pork generously with the olive oil mixture, and spread with barbecue sauce.
- Place string beans around the pork in the slow cooker.
- Cook for 7-8 hours on low.

Nutrition facts per serving **(215 g)**
Calories: 472
Total fat: 5.3 g
Carbohydrates: 75.8 g
Dietary fiber: 2.3 g
Sugars: 40.6 g
Protein: 28.5 g

Creamy Cheesy Turkey Casserole

Servings: 4
Preparation time: 10 minutes
Cooking time: 5 hours

Ingredients:
1 pound fresh turkey, thinly sliced
1 15 oz. can lima beans
1 cup cream cheese
2 tomatoes, diced
1 6 oz. can tomato paste
1 teaspoon black pepper, ground
Salt

Directions:
- Place turkey, lima beans, tomatoes, tomato paste, and black pepper in the slow cooker. Season with salt to taste.
- Cook for 4 hours on low.
- Stir in the cream cheese and cook for 1 more hour.
- Serve with a baked potato or rice.

Nutrition facts per serving (490 g)
Calories: 675
Total fat: 34.0 g
Carbohydrates: 51.0 g
Dietary fiber: 12.1 g
Sugars: 8.9 g
Protein: 47.8 g

Cheese and Beef Meatballs

Servings: 4-6
Preparation time: 15 minutes
Cooking time: 7 hours

Ingredients:
20 gluten-free frozen beef meat balls
2 tablespoons olive oil
1 6 oz. can of tomato paste
1 cup tomato sauce
2 teaspoons chili powder
2 teaspoons paprika
1 cup beef broth
¾ cup grated cheddar cheese

Directions:
- Sprinkle black pepper over the meatballs.
- Place the meatballs, olive oil, tomato paste, tomato sauce, chili powder, paprika powder, and broth in slow cooker.
- Cook for 6 hours on low.
- Sprinkle cheddar cheese on top and cook for 1 more hour.

Nutrition facts per serving (230 g)
Calories: 705
Total fat: 23.0 g
Carbohydrates: 83.7 g
Dietary fiber: 3.2 g
Sugars: 3.6 g
Protein: 37.2 g

Juicy Lamb Chops

Servings: 4-6
Preparation time: 30 minutes
Cooking time: 12 hours

Ingredients:
2 pounds lamb chops, cut in 1 ½ inch chops
2 tablespoons vegetable oil
2 tablespoons black pepper, ground
2 tablespoons black pepper, whole
½ teaspoon salt
¼ cup onion, chopped
¼ cup garlic, minced
2 tablespoons oregano, ground
2 tablespoons mustard seeds, ground
1 cup vegetable or chicken broth
½ cup gluten-free soy sauce

Directions:
- Rub lamb with salt and ground pepper. Arrange in the slow cooker.
- Combine the oil, whole black pepper, onion, garlic, oregano, mustard seeds, broth and soy sauce, and add.
- Cook for 12 hours on a low setting.
- Serve with steamed rice and salad.

***Nutrition facts per serving* (627 g)**
Calories: 627
Total fat: 32.7 g
Carbohydrates: 26.1 g
Dietary fiber: 2.6 g
Sugars: 5.6 g
Protein: 127.6 g

Korean-Style Honeyed Chicken

Servings: 4
Preparation time: 1 hour
Cooking time: 10 hours

Ingredients:
1 whole chicken, about 5-6 pounds
2 teaspoons sea salt
4 teaspoons turmeric, ground
4 teaspoons chili powder
4 teaspoons black pepper, ground
¼ cup onion, diced
½ cup garlic, minced
3 tablespoons honey
¼ cup brown sugar
2 tablespoons olive or vegetable oil

Directions:
- Mix the salt, turmeric, chili powder, black pepper, and brown sugar in a small bowl. Rub the chicken skin with the mixture.
- Spread the oil over the bottom of the slow cooker. Place the chicken breast-side up in the slow cooker and surround with onion, garlic, and honey.
- Cook for 10 hours on low.
- Check to ensure that the chicken is cooked. The juice should run clear when poked with a fork in the thigh. The temperature on a meat thermometer should read 165ºF when inserted in the thickest part of the breast without touching any bones.

Note: you can add some peeled potatoes and carrots after 5 hours of cooking to make the chicken a one pot meal. If the bottom of the slow cooker is too dry just add a bit of water or chicken stock before adding the vegetables.

Nutrition facts per serving **(195 g)**
Calories: 328
Total fat: 25.4 g
Carbohydrates: 3.4 g
Dietary fiber: 0.9 g
Sugars: 30.3 g
Protein: 28.5 g

Turkey Soda Roast

Servings: 6
Preparation time: 10 minutes
Cooking time: 8 hours

Ingredients:
3 pounds whole fresh turkey breast
1 can lemon soda, such as 7-Up™ or Mountain Dew™
1½ cup chicken or vegetable broth
1 small yellow onion, diced
1 tablespoon black peppercorns
¼ cup mushrooms, sliced
¼ cup butter, melted
1 teaspoon smoked paprika
½ teaspoon of salt
½ teaspoon of pepper, ground

Directions:
- Place turkey in the slow cooker, and brush with the melted butter. Season with paprika.
- Carefully pour the soda and broth around the turkey, and add the onions, mushrooms, and whole black pepper. Season with salt and freshly ground black pepper.
- Cook for 8 hours on a low setting.

Nutrition facts per serving (380 g)
Calories: 692
Total fat: 40.1 g
Carbohydrates: 10.2 g
Dietary fiber: 0.2 g
Sugars: 6.2 g
Protein: 65.5 g

Creamy Corn and Pork Bits

Servings: 8
Preparation time: 15 minutes
Cooking time: 7 hours

Ingredients:
2 pounds ground pork
1 ½ cups corn kernels, frozen or canned
1 cup milk
½ cup sour cream, plus extra for serving
5 teaspoons butter, melted
1 tablespoon honey
2 tablespoons fresh chives, chopped (or 1 tablespoon dried chives)
Salt and pepper

Directions:
- Place ground pork in a skillet and brown. Drain the fat.
- Add the pork to the slow cooker, and add the corn, milk, sour cream, butter, honey, and chives.
- Set the slow cooker to low and cook for 7 hours.
- Top with a dollop of sour cream before serving.

Nutrition facts per serving (225 g)
Calories: 248
Total fat: 8.5 g
Carbohydrates: 42.3 g
Dietary fiber: 4.8 g
Sugars: 0.9 g
Protein: 6.8 g

Peppery Creamy Chicken

Servings: 6

Preparation time: 6 minutes
Cooking time: 6 hours

Ingredients:
2 pounds skinless chicken breasts, about 6
2 tablespoons olive oil
1 cup chicken broth
2 teaspoons black pepper, ground
1 tablespoon black pepper peppercorn, whole
½ cup sour cream
4 tablespoons butter, melted
1 bunch of fresh parsley, chopped
Steamed brown or white rice for serving

Directions:
- In the slow cooker, layer the olive oil, chicken, chicken broth, ground black pepper and whole black pepper. Cook on a low setting for 4 hours.
- Stir in sour cream, butter, and parsley. Cook for 2 more hours.
- Serve with one cup of steamed rice.

Nutrition facts per serving (175 g)*
Calories: 344
Total fat: 23.7 g
Carbohydrates: 6.7 g
Dietary fiber: 1.7 g
Sugars: 3.2 g
Protein: 30.6 g
* without rice

Honey Mustard Pork Slices

Servings: 4
Preparation time: 15 minutes
Cooking time: 4 hours

Ingredients:
2 pounds pork tenderloin, sliced thinly
2 teaspoons black pepper, ground
1 teaspoon salt
¼ cup mustard
2 tablespoons mustard seeds, ground
2 tablespoons honey
½ cup balsamic vinegar
2 teaspoons black pepper, ground

Directions:
- Rub pork with black pepper and salt.
- In slow cooker, arrange prepared pork, mustard, mustard seeds, honey, balsamic vinegar, and black pepper.
- Cook for 4 hours on a high setting.
- Serve with steamed rice or baked potato.

Nutrition facts per serving (184 g)
Calories: 138
Total fat: 7.8 g
Carbohydrates: 7.7 g
Dietary fiber: 0.7 g
Sugars: 5.6 g
Protein: 9.1 g

Pork Chops and Buttered Vegetables

Servings: 4
Preparation time: 10 minutes
Cooking time: 7 hours

Ingredients:
4-6 pork chops
¼ cup onion, chopped
¼ cup garlic, minced
1 bunch of parsley, chopped
¼ cup of green bell pepper, diced
¼ cup of red bell pepper, diced
1 cup tomatoes, diced
1 tablespoon black peppercorns, whole
¼ cup butter
1 cup green peas
1 cup carrots, diced
1 cup butternut squash, diced
1 cup corn kernels

Directions:
- Arrange the pork chops in the slow cooker, and add the onion, garlic, parsley, green bell pepper, red bell pepper, tomatoes and whole peppercorns.
- Cook for 7 hours on low.
- Melt the butter in a medium skillet, and lightly fry the green peas, carrots, butternut squash, and corn.
- Serve pork chops together with buttered vegetables and rice.

Nutrition facts per serving **(494 g)**
Calories: 483
Total fat: 18.4 g
Carbohydrates: 35.8 g
Dietary fiber: 3.4 g
Sugars: 22.2 g
Protein: 44.2 g

Vegetable and Legume Stew

Servings: 6
Preparation time: 15 minutes
Cooking time: 12 hours

Ingredients:
1 28-oz. can kidney beans, rinsed and drained
1 28 oz. can black-eye beans, rinsed and drained
1 cup carrots, diced
1 cup celery, diced
1 cup potatoes, diced
1 small onions, diced
4 garlic cloves, minced
1 tablespoon dried oregano
1 tablespoon ground rosemary
1 tablespoon black pepper, ground
1 tablespoon paprika
4 cups vegetable or chicken broth
1 cup water

Directions:
- In the slow cooker, mix kidney beans, mongo beans, carrots, potatoes, onions, garlic, oregano, rosemary, black pepper, paprika, broth, and water.
- Cook for 10-12 hours on low.
- Serve with gluten-free bread or crackers.

***Nutrition facts per serving* (258 g)**
Calories: 164
Total fat: 0.5 g
Carbohydrates: 32.3 g
Dietary fiber: 12.7 g
Sugars: 6.2 g
Protein: 10.4

Chili Salmon Fillets

Servings: 8
Preparation time: 15 minutes
Cooking time: 7 hours

Ingredients:
4 salmon fillets, about 8 oz. each
2 tablespoons olive oil
¼ cup minced garlic
¼ cup onion, chopped
1 cup kidney beans, rinsed and drained
½ cup red bell pepper, diced
½ cup green bell pepper, diced
1 cup tomatoes, diced
1 cup tomato sauce
3 teaspoons chili powder
1 teaspoon ground cumin

Directions:
- Sauté salmon fillets, olive oil, and onion for 8-10 minutes. Add the garlic, and stir until fragrant.
- Place cooked salmon fillets into the slow cooker with kidney beans, red bell pepper, green bell pepper, tomatoes, tomato sauce, chili powder, and cumin.
- Cook for 7 hours on low.
- Serve with baked potatoes or steamed rice.

Nutrition facts per serving **(416 g)**

Calories: 293
Total fat: 2.7 g
Carbohydrates: 58.3 g
Dietary fiber: 15.3 g
Sugars: 12.5 g
Protein: 14.9 g

Cheesy Beef Ravioli

Servings: 6-8
Preparation time: 10 minutes
Cooking time: 5 hours

Ingredients:

1 package of gluten-free ravioli, about 25-30 oz.
2 cups ground beef
1 tablespoon oregano, ground
1 tablespoon Spanish paprika
¼ cup butter, melted
1 cup tomatoes, diced
1 cup tomato paste
1 cup vegetable or beef broth
½ cup red bell pepper, diced
½ cup green bell pepper, diced
1 cup mozzarella cheese

Directions:

- In a medium skillet, crumble the ground beef and fry until browned. Drain the fat and season with oregano and Spanish paprika.
- In the slow cooker, mix the ground beef, butter, tomatoes, tomato paste, broth, red bell pepper, and green bell pepper.
- Cook for 3 hours on high.
- Add ravioli and mozzarella cheese and cook for 2 more hours.

Nutrition facts per serving **(289 g)**
Calories: 487
Total fat: 27.9 g
Carbohydrates: 38.6 g
Dietary fiber: 4.2 g
Sugars: 14.1 g
Protein: 7.1 g

DESSERT RECIPES

Vanilla and Honey Bananas

Servings: 4
Preparation time: 10 minutes
Cooking time: 1 hour

Ingredients:
5 bananas, sliced
1 teaspoon vanilla extract
1 tablespoon honey
5 tablespoons brown sugar
½ cup condensed milk
½ cup evaporated milk
½ cup milk powder
Chocolate syrup

Directions:
- In a slow cooker, gently mix sliced bananas, vanilla extract, honey, brown sugar, condensed milk, evaporated milk and milk powder.
- Cook for 1 hour on a low setting.
- Serve with chocolate syrup.

Nutrition facts per serving (232 g)
Calories: 343
Total fat: 11.8 g
Carbohydrates: 55.0 g
Dietary fiber: 4.5 g
Sugars: 34.8 g
Protein: 2.1 g

Cinnamon Pears

Servings: 4
Preparation time: 30 minutes
Cooking time: 2 hours

Ingredients:
5 pears, sliced into two
2 teaspoons of cinnamon
1 teaspoon nutmeg
2 tablespoons honey
4 tablespoons brown sugar

Directions:
- In a slow cooker, combine the pears, cinnamon, nutmeg, honey, and brown sugar.
- Cook for 2 hours on high.
- Sprinkle with more cinnamon before serving.

Nutrition facts per serving (302 g)
Calories: 658
Total fat: 13.3 g
Carbohydrates: 144.5 g
Dietary fiber: 11.5 g
Sugars: 118.5 g
Protein: 2.4 g

Spiced Up Veggies with Apples

Servings: 8-10
Preparation time: 45 minutes
Cooking time: 6 hours

Ingredients:
5 cups cabbage, shredded
½ cup onion, diced
4 cups of apples, diced
2 teaspoons chili powder
2 tablespoons honey
3 tablespoons brown sugar
1 teaspoon cinnamon
1 teaspoon black pepper, ground
4 tablespoons balsamic vinegar
Salt and pepper

Directions:
- In a slow cooker, combine cabbage, onion, apples, chili powder, honey, brown sugar, cinnamon, black pepper, and balsamic vinegar.
- Cook for 6 hours on a low setting.
- Season with salt and pepper before serving.

Nutrition facts per serving (253 g)
Calories: 178
Total fat: 3.3 g
Carbohydrates: 39.1 g
Dietary fiber: 6.9 g
Sugars: 25.6 g
Protein: 2.8 g

Strawberry Fudge Slices

Servings: 6
Preparation time: 25 minutes
Cooking time: 3 hours

Ingredients:
2 cups strawberries, hulled and quartered
¼ cup brown sugar
2 tablespoons honey
1 cup of milk chocolate, melted
4 tablespoons butter, melted
2 teaspoons gluten-free cornstarch

Directions:
- Place at the bottom of the slow cooker the melted butter, then the corn starch, then the milk chocolate.
- Cook for 1 hour on a high setting.
- Add in the strawberries, honey, and brown sugar.
- Cook for 2 hours on a high setting.
- Cool until set. Slice into desired sizes before serving.

Nutrition facts per serving (2168 g)
Calories: 223
Total fat: 0.8 g
Carbohydrates: 59.7 g
Dietary fiber: 7.4 g
Sugars: 48.2 g
Protein: 0.9 g

Caramel Apples

Servings: 4-5
Preparation time: 20 minutes
Cooking time: 3 hours

Ingredients:
4 apples, halved and cored
½ cup raisins
½ cup mixed nuts, ground
½ cup brown sugar
2 tablespoons honey
1 teaspoon cinnamon
½ teaspoon salt
Vanilla ice cream

Directions:
- Place brown sugar and honey in the slow cooker.
- Cook for 1 hour on low.
- Add in the apples, raisins, mixed nuts, cinnamon, and salt.
- Cook for 2 more hours.
- Serve with vanilla ice cream.

Nutrition facts per serving (215 g)
Calories: 479
Total fat: 22.7 g
Carbohydrates: 78.2 g
Dietary fiber: 6.7 g
Sugars: 68.0 g
Protein: 1.9 g

Almond Chocolate Drink

Servings: 12
Preparation time: 5 minutes
Cooking time: 2 hours

Ingredients:
1 cup gluten-free semi-sweet chocolate chips
¼ cup almonds, ground
2 cups milk
2 teaspoons nutmeg
1 teaspoon honey
Whipped cream

Directions:
- In a slow cooker chocolate chunks, ground almonds, milk, and nutmeg.
- Cook for 2 hours on low.
- Serve with whipped cream.

Nutrition facts per serving (164 g)
Calories: 161
Total fat: 12.3 g
Carbohydrates: 9.4 g
Dietary fiber: 0.0 g
Sugars: 5.5 g
Protein: 6.0 g

Pineapple Gluten-Free Bread Pudding

Servings: 6
Preparation time: 15 minutes
Cooking time: 6 hours

Ingredients:
1 cup pineapple, chopped into bite-sized chunks
3 tablespoons butter, melted
1 cup milk
¼ cup condensed milk
¼ cup brown sugar
1 tablespoon lemon juice
8 gluten-free bread slices, cut into cubes
3 eggs
1 teaspoon cinnamon

Directions:
- In the slow cooker, place butter, milk, condensed milk and brown sugar. Whip the eggs and place in the bottom layer too.
- Layer in the gluten-free bread slices then cook for 2 hours.
- Add the pineapples, lemon juice, and cinnamon.
- Cook for 4 hours on low.
- Slice into desired sizes.

Nutrition facts per serving **(225 g)**
Calories: 547
Total fat: 17.2 g
Carbohydrates: 86.5 g
Dietary fiber: 2.5 g
Sugars: 49.2 g
Protein: 13.3 g

S'mores Squares

Servings: 2-3
Preparation time: 15 minutes
Cooking time: 4 hours

Ingredients:
3 cups marshmallows
1 cup milk
¼ cup condensed milk
¼ cup brown sugar
1 tablespoon lemon juice
1 cup gluten-free chocolate pieces (milk or dark), cut into chunks
1 cup gluten-free rice crackers, crushed
¼ cup butter, melted

Directions:
- Pour melted butter into the slow cooker and add crushed rice crackers, milk, condensed milk, brown sugar, and lemon juice.
- Sprinkle the marshmallows and chocolate pieces on top.
- Cook for 4 hours on a low setting.

***Nutrition facts per serving* (180 g)**
Calories: 250
Total fat: 38.5 g
Carbohydrates: 48.1 g
Dietary fiber: 1.3 g
Sugars: 59.5 g
Protein: 0.9 g

CONCLUSION

Living gluten-free can be overwhelming when it comes to food preparation. Using your slow cooker makes it so much easier. You get great tasting food, one pot meal, and an easy clean up!.

So there you have it, the simplest way to live gluten-free with these easy to prepare and stress-free one pot meals your family will love. I hope you found several to add to your go-to recipes Thank you so much for downloading and reading my book.

Notes

Made in the USA
San Bernardino, CA
17 December 2018